Back on Track

Heal and Prevent Back Pain Naturally

Harmony Royce

DEDICATION

To people who are dedicated to getting better and leading pain-free lives, as well as to those who have battled back pain. I hope that this book will be a helpful resource that gives you the courage and information to take charge of your health in addition to providing you with relief.

To my family, friends, and supporters, who have always inspired me with their support and faith in me. I appreciate your steadfast support.

And this book is for everyone who is prepared to start the healing process.

DISCLAIMER

Back on Track: Heal and Prevent Back Pain Naturally contains information that is meant only for educational reasons and should not be used in place of expert medical advice, diagnosis, or treatment. Although the techniques and approaches covered in this book are supported by credible research and professional advice, individual outcomes may differ. Before beginning any new therapy, treatment, or workout regimen, always get medical advice, especially if you have any pre-existing health issues.

Any harm, loss, or damage resulting from the use or implementation of the material in this book is not the responsibility of the author or publisher. You accept complete responsibility for your personal health and well-being by using the material given.

CONTENTS

ACKNOWLEDGMENTS

Without the assistance and efforts of numerous people, this book would not have been possible. I am extremely appreciative of the medical professionals, therapists, and specialists whose skills and knowledge have influenced the substance of my work. Their observations have guaranteed that the data presented is correct, useful, and based on the most recent studies.

I also want to express my gratitude to the several people who have contributed their own tales and experiences of dealing with back pain. Your bravery, candor, and desire to help have been crucial in influencing and motivating the writing of this book.

Thank you to the enthusiastic and trusting readers who make up this supportive group. This work is driven by your commitment to bettering your health, and I hope it helps you on your path to pain management and long-term wellbeing.

Finally, I would like to express my sincere gratitude to

everyone who has supported and believed in our initiative, which has helped make this book a reality. This effort has been made possible by your support.

CHAPTER 1

UNDERSTANDING BACK PAIN

Millions of people worldwide suffer from back discomfort, which is a common problem. Despite its widespread occurrence, people frequently fail to adequately address it due to a lack of knowledge, stigma, and misunderstanding. This chapter delves deeply into the widespread myths, the wide-ranging effects, and the complex structure of the spine, giving readers the fundamental knowledge they need to understand and treat back pain more effectively.

1.1 Typical Myths Regarding Back Pain

Many people have misconceptions regarding back pain, which are fueled by out-of-date advice and simplistic ideas. Let's examine the consequences of some of the most common myths and dispel them:

Myth: The Best Cure Is Rest

Long-term inactivity can make back pain worse, even though rest is crucial during its acute phase. This is the reason:

- Deconditioning: Prolonged periods of inactivity weaken the back and core muscles that support the spine, which makes the body less stable and more prone to injury.

- **Stiffness and Reduced Mobility:** Insufficient mobility can lead to stiff spinal joints, which can make daily tasks more difficult and uncomfortable.

- Psychological Effects: Chronic pain syndromes and emotions of helplessness are frequently exacerbated by inactivity.

Modern Perspective: Low-impact exercises, such as yoga or swimming, physical therapy, and leading an active lifestyle are increasingly regarded as crucial elements of healing.

Myth: Injury Is Always the Cause of Back Pain

Back pain is not always caused by a specific injury or event, despite what many people think. Numerous non-injury-related causes may be included, such as:

- **Bad Posture:** Long-term improper sitting or standing posture can put stress on the spine.

- **Lifestyle Decisions:** Sedentary living, smoking, and obesity are major risk factors.

- **Degenerative Conditions:** Degenerative disc disease and osteoarthritis are two age-related conditions that frequently cause back discomfort without any obvious "injury."

- **Stress:** Tension in the muscles brought on by emotional stress can result in pain and chronic discomfort.

Observation: Managing underlying medical issues and lifestyle choices might be just as important as treating physical injuries.

Myth: The Only Way to Fix It Is Through Surgery

Although surgery is frequently thought of as the only option for people with severe back pain, it is not always required or even advised. Think about the following:

- Acupuncture, physical therapy, chiropractic adjustments, and mindfulness-based interventions are examples of non-surgical alternatives that can offer significant relief.

- **Dangers and Restrictions of Surgery:** Surgical procedures like disc replacement or spinal fusion are susceptible to infection, a protracted recuperation period, or even unsatisfactory results.

- **Progress in Pain Management:** Non-surgical methods that work include nerve blocks, epidural steroid injections, and regenerative medicine (such as platelet-rich plasma therapy).

Details: Generally speaking, surgery should only be performed after conservative measures have failed or when certain disorders, such severe spinal stenosis, call for it.

1.2 Back Pain's Prevalence and Effects

Comprehending the extent and consequences of back pain highlights its importance as a worldwide health concern.

Global Statistics

- The Global Burden of Disease Study indicates that back pain is the leading cause of disability worldwide.

- At some point in their life, about 80% of adults will suffer from back discomfort.

- Every year, the illness costs billions of dollars in medical expenses and missed productivity.

Workplace Implications

- **Absenteeism:** One of the main reasons for missing work days is back pain. This problem results in the loss of more than **264 million workdays per year** in the United States alone.

- **Decreased Productivity:** Workers with persistent back discomfort frequently report being less focused and producing less.

- **Claims for Workers' Compensation:** The ailment is one of the most commonly reported causes of job injuries.

Emotional Cost

Beyond only being physically uncomfortable, chronic back pain frequently results in:

- **Anxiety and Depression:** The ongoing nature of pain can have an impact on mental health.

- Feelings of loneliness might result from limited

movement, which makes it difficult to engage in social activities.

- **Sleep Disruptions:** Pain often prevents people from getting a good night's sleep, which exacerbates emotional stress and exhaustion.

Call to Action: Prioritizing prevention, early intervention, and comprehensive treatment requires an understanding of the wide-ranging effects of back pain.

1.3 The Spine's Anatomy

The spine, which supports the body, allows for mobility, and shields the central nervous system, is a marvel of biological engineering.

Overview of Structure

There are four sections to the human spine:

1. The neck, or cervical spine, is made up of seven vertebrae (C1–C7). This area allows for a great range of mobility and supports the head.

2. Comprising 12 vertebrae (T1–T12), the thoracic spine (upper back) attaches to the rib cage and

stabilizes and protects critical organs.

3. **Lumbar Spine (Lower Back):** Made up of five vertebrae (L1-L5), it is prone to damage and supports the majority of the body's weight.

4. The sacrum, which consists of five fused vertebrae, and the coccyx, which is the tailbone, comprise the base of the spine and provide structural support.

Primary Elements

- **Vertebrae:** The separate bones that make up the spine.

- Intervertebral discs are gel-like cushions that provide flexibility and shock absorption between vertebrae.

- The little joints at the rear of the spine that allow for smooth movement are called facet joints.

- **Spinal Cord and Nerves:** Nerves branch out from the spinal cord, which passes through the vertebral canal, to transmit information from the brain to the body.

How It Operates

A fine balance between strength and flexibility is made possible by the spine's biomechanics:

- **Weight Distribution:** The cervical spine provides flexibility for head movement, while the lumbar spine is specifically designed to support large weights.

- **Extension and Flexion:** The structure of the spinal column permits twisting as well as forward, backward, and sideways bending.

- The absorption of shock: As shock absorbers, intervertebral discs shield the spine from harm when engaging in high-impact activities.

Common Vulnerabilities:

- **Wear and Tear:** Because of its weight-bearing function, the lumbar region is particularly vulnerable to degenerative disorders.

- **Inadequate mechanics:** Injuries may result from bad posture or from lifting large objects.

Result: Recognizing the causes of back pain and putting effective preventive measures in place require a thorough understanding of spinal structure.

Back pain is a complex problem with significant social,

emotional, and physical ramifications. The foundation for addressing this widespread ailment is laid by debunking myths, comprehending its prevalence, and recognizing the intricate structure of the spine. We can open the door to improved care, prevention, and general spinal health by arming people with factual information.

CHAPTER 2

THE FUNDAMENTALS OF MECHANICAL BACK PAIN

One of the most prevalent and poorly understood sources of discomfort, mechanical back pain affects people of all ages. In addition to understanding the complex interactions between spinal discs and nerve pathways, this chapter offers a thorough examination of its nature, causes, and manifestations.

2.1 Mechanical Back Pain: What Is It?

Explanation

The term "mechanical back pain" describes pain that comes from the spine, intervertebral discs, muscles, or ligaments as opposed to being brought on by an infection, inflammatory disease, or systemic illness. This kind of discomfort is frequently localized and usually affected by movement. It differs from diseases with various underlying processes, such as neuropathic pain or inflammatory arthritis.

Triggers

Biomechanical tension or strain is the main cause of mechanical back pain. Typical triggers consist of:

- The lumbar and cervical spines are strained when people slouch or sit for long periods of time.
- Micro-injuries can develop over time as a result of improper spinal alignment during normal activities.

Improper Lifting Techniques:

- The lower back is overworked while bending at the waist rather than the knees.
- Acute injuries might result from twisting when lifting big objects.

Repetitive Strain:

- Activities that require bending, twisting, or lifting repeatedly can harm muscles, ligaments, and joints over time.
- Jobs that need a lot of standing or sitting also increase the risk of repetitive strain injuries.

Symptoms

Recognizing important traits is necessary to diagnose

mechanical back pain:

- The lumbar region of the lower back is a common location for localized pain, which is made worse by movement.

- **Stiffness:** Joint stiffness or tense muscles make it difficult to bend or rotate the spine.

- **Pain Relief with Rest:** Rest or a change in posture usually relieves symptoms.

- **Lack of Systemic Symptoms**: Fever, severe weight loss, or exhaustion are not associated with mechanical back pain, in contrast to inflammatory or viral causes.

Primary Finding: The development of chronic back pain can be avoided by identifying and treating the causes of mechanical back pain early on.

2.2 Comprehending Health and Disc Function

The unsung heroes of spinal health are the intervertebral discs. These structures are essential for protecting the spine, preserving flexibility, and absorbing shocks.

Discs' role

Each of the 23 intervertebral discs in the spine serves as a cushion between neighboring vertebrae. Among their roles are:

- The impact of everyday movements like walking, running, and leaping is absorbed by the discs.
- They enable the spine to bend, twist, and stretch without making contact with other bones.
- **Load Distribution:** Discs lessen wear and tear by distributing the body's weight evenly across the spinal column.

Degenerative Problems

- **Disc degeneration** is the term used to describe the natural changes that occur in the intervertebral discs as we age. Important elements consist of:

Disc Dehydration:

- A gel-like, water-rich nucleus pulposus is found in healthy discs. Discs lose moisture with time, which lessens their capacity to cushion.
- Less intervertebral space may result from the thinning and bulging of degenerated discs.
- Neurological problems and pain may result from

bulging discs pressing on nearby nerves.

Herniated Discs:

- The nucleus pulposus can irritate neighboring nerves when it pokes through the outer layer (annulus fibrosus).

Warning Signs Disc-related problems frequently coexist with mechanical back pain, although they can also include:

- **Persistent Pain:** Particularly after standing or sitting for extended periods of time.
- Radiating pain, which is frequently observed in sciatica, is pain that radiates to the arms, legs, or buttocks.
- **Numbness or weakness:** These signs suggest that nerves may be affected.
- **Decreased Flexibility:** Pain or stiffness that makes it difficult to bend or twist.

Result: The chance of developing mechanical back pain can be considerably decreased by maintaining disc health through exercise, good posture, and hydration.

2.3 Nerve Involvement and Pain Pathways

Different levels of discomfort are caused by nerve irritation or compression, which is a common component of mechanical back pain experience. Effective diagnosis and treatment depend on an understanding of these pain pathways.

Compression of Nerves

The spinal cord, which supplies the rest of the body with nerve roots, is located in the spine. Pain or other neurological symptoms may arise from the compression or pinching of these nerves:

Consistent Causes:

- **Bulging or herniated discs.**
- A narrowing of the spinal canal is known as spinal stenosis.
- Nerve roots affected by osteoarthritis or bone spurs.

The following are signs of nerve compression:

- Localized soreness in the back.
- Pain that travels down the arms or legs.
- Weakness, numbness, or tingling in the extremities.

Symptoms of Radiation

- Pain radiating along the nerve's route is one of the classic signs of nerve involvement.

- Compression of the sciatic nerve results in sciatica, which causes pain, tingling, or paralysis in the legs, buttocks, and lower back.

- Prolonged sitting, coughing, or sneezing might exacerbate it.

Cervical Radiculopathy:

- Compression of the cervical spine's nerves can result in numbness, weakness, or arm pain.

Comprehending Pain Signals

Two categories can be used to describe how the body reacts to pain:

Acute Pain:

- Occurs unexpectedly, frequently as a result of trauma.

- It acts as a safeguard, alerting the body to possible danger.

- Usually goes away after the underlying problem is addressed.

Chronic Pain:

- It frequently lasts longer than the typical recovery period, lasting longer than three months.
- Sensitization of pain pathways may occur, causing severe agony in response to even small stimuli.
- Chronic pain can be exacerbated by psychological conditions including depression and anxiety.

Managing Pain Pathways:

- Acute mechanical pain is frequently relieved by non-invasive therapies such as stretching, physical therapy, and ergonomic adjustments.
- Interventions include spinal cord stimulation, nerve blocks, and cognitive behavioral therapy (CBT) can help control symptoms of long-term illnesses.

Despite being widespread, mechanical back pain is a complex ailment that necessitates a sophisticated comprehension of its roots and consequences. People can take proactive measures toward prevention and treatment by distinguishing it from other forms of pain, identifying its origins and symptoms, and comprehending the role of spinal discs and nerve involvement. Equipped with this understanding, patients and medical professionals can work together to create individualized treatment plans for improved spine health.

together to create individualized treatment plans for improved spine health.

CHAPTER 3

Typical Back Pain Causes

Back pain has several underlying causes and is a worldwide health concern. By exploring the most common causes, such as bad posture, lifestyle choices, and physical injuries, this chapter offers a thorough grasp of their effects as well as practical ways to lessen them.

3.1 Bad Body Language

Impact of Modern Lifestyle

As more people work at desks and spend more time on screens, bad posture is now the main cause of back discomfort. Long-term use of non-ergonomic seating arrangements might result in:

- **Muscle Imbalances:** As time passes, certain muscles (like the core stabilizers) weaken while others (like the hip flexors) become hyperactive.

- An example of spinal misalignment is Leaning

forward or slouching alters the natural curves of the spine, putting more strain on the intervertebral discs.

- **Persistent Tension:** Poor posture can cause shoulder and neck strains, which can result in upper back pain.

The use of ergonomic solutions

Back discomfort brought on by poor posture can be lessened by using ergonomics both at work and at home.

Important suggestions consist of:

Chair Adjustment:

- Make use of a chair that supports your lumbar region.
- To keep your spine neutral, make sure your hips are a little higher than your knees.

Desk Setup:

- To avoid neck strain, place the monitor at eye level.
- To prevent overextension, keep the mouse and keyboard close at hand.

Standing Desks:

- To lessen extended strain on the spine, alternate between sitting and standing.

Awareness of Posture

For long-term treatment, it is essential to include posture-promoting exercises. Among the examples are:

- **Wall Angels:** To increase shoulder mobility, stand up against a wall and slowly raise and lower your arms while maintaining contact with the wall.

- **Cat-Cow Stretch:** To improve spinal alignment and flexibility, alternate between rounding and arching your back.

- Exercises that strengthen the core, such as bird-dogs and planks, help to stabilize the spine and lessen the strain on nearby tissues.

Primary Finding: Chronic back pain can be considerably decreased by being aware of one's daily posture and making proactive adjustments.

3.2 Causes Associated with Lifestyle

Obesity: Excess weight puts more mechanical strain on the spine, especially in the lumbar area. Among the repercussions are:

- Excess weight accelerates degeneration by

compressing intervertebral discs, resulting in increased disc pressure.

- **Altered Spinal Curves:** Anterior pelvic tilt brought on by obesity might result in increased lumbar lordosis (swayback).

- **Joint Wear and Tear:** The extra strain encourages osteoarthritis in the spinal joints to develop early.

Solutions:

- **Weight Management:** To lessen the strain on the spine, including regular activity and a healthy diet.

- **Activities with Little Impact:** Walking and swimming reduce spinal strain and help people lose weight.

Sedentary Behavior: The muscles supporting the spine get weaker with inactivity, increasing the likelihood of pain. Important concerns include:

- **Decreased Flexibility:** Extended periods of inactivity can cause tight muscles and stiff joints, which limit mobility.

- Inactivity is associated with systemic inflammation, which exacerbates discomfort.

- **Muscle Atrophy:** Absence of use reduces muscle strength, especially in the lower back and core.

Solutions:

- Regular Movement Breaks: Stretch and exercise for five to ten minutes every hour.
- Regular exercise, such as yoga, pilates, or tai chi, can help you become more flexible and strong.

Health of the Spine and Smoking

Smoking's impacts on spinal health make it a lesser-known but important cause of back pain. Important mechanisms consist of:

- **Decreased Oxygen Supply:** Smoking accelerates degeneration by reducing blood flow to the spinal discs.
- **Weakened Bone Health:** Nicotine reduces bone density and increases the risk of fracture by interfering with calcium absorption.
- Smokers' poorer recovery from back injuries is a result of their reduced ability to repair damaged tissue.

Solutions:

- **Smoking Cessation:** Use nicotine replacement therapy or look for assistance from smoking cessation programs.

- **Bone Health Assistance:** To reverse the effects of smoking on bone density, make sure you are getting enough calcium and vitamin D.

Result: Making lifestyle changes is essential to lowering the incidence and severity of back pain.

3.3 Overuse and Traumatic Injuries

Injuries From Lifting

Acute back discomfort is frequently brought on by improper lifting techniques, especially at work. Common errors include carrying too-heavy goods, twisting when lifting, and bending at the waist. Ligament sprains, disc herniation, and muscular strains are among the consequences.

Preventive Advice:

- **Lift with Your Legs:** Maintain a straight back while

lifting and bend at the knees.

- **Keep the Load near:** Reducing the amount of strain on your spine can be achieved by holding objects near to your body.
- **Avoid Twisting:** Instead of twisting your torso, pivot with your feet.

Strength Associated with Sports

Because of overtraining, impact, and repeated actions, athletes and leisure sports fans are more likely to have back pain. Typical actions that could be involved include:

- Running and gymnastics are examples of high-impact sports that put repetitive pressure on the spine.
- **Sports that rotate:** Tennis and golf require repetitive twisting motions, which can result in overuse problems.
- **Sports Contact:** Traumatic spine injuries are more likely to occur in sports like rugby and football.

Preventive Advice:

- **Adequate Warm-Up:** Always use dynamic stretching to get joints and muscles ready for action.

- To improve stability and lessen strain during sports, strengthen your core muscles with strength training.

- **Rest and Recovery:** Make sure to schedule enough days off so that the body may recuperate from strenuous activity.

Repeated Motions

Overuse injuries can result from repetitive motion-intensive jobs and pastimes including gardening and assembly line work. These happen when tissues experience repeated stress without sufficient recuperation.

The danger is increased when repetitive tasks are performed in awkward positions due to poor ergonomics.

- **Inadequate Rest:** Uninterrupted activity hinders the healing of tissues.

Mitigation Strategies:

- **Modify Techniques:** To reduce strain, use tools or modify body mechanics.

- **Take Regular Breaks:** Stop often to relax and stretch strained muscles.

Primary Finding: To preserve long-term spinal health, traumatic and overuse injuries must be recognized and prevented.

Despite being widespread, back discomfort frequently results from preventable causes. Its occurrence is greatly increased by bad posture, harmful lifestyle choices, and physical injuries. People can lower their chance of experiencing back pain and enhance their general quality of life by being aware of these factors and putting preventive measures in place, such as ergonomic changes, weight management, regular exercise, and safe lifting practices. Giving them this information lays the groundwork for long-term health and proactive spinal care.

CHAPTER 4

STRATEGIES FOR PREVENTION

A multimodal strategy that incorporates stress management strategies, workplace modifications, and healthy lifestyle choices is needed to prevent back discomfort. This chapter examines practical methods for preserving spinal health and reducing the likelihood of back discomfort, with a focus on long-term habits that fit in well with everyday life.

4.1 Modifications to Lifestyle

Nutrition for Spine Health: Dietary Considerations

Strong bones, good intervertebral discs, and general spinal integrity are all dependent on proper nutrition. Important dietary considerations are:

- Vitamin D and calcium are necessary for strong and dense bones. Dairy products, leafy greens, and fortified foods are examples of sources. Vitamin D synthesis is increased by exposure to sunlight.

- **Foods that reduce inflammation:** Incorporating foods high in omega-3 fatty acids (such as fish, walnuts, and flaxseed), antioxidants (such as berries and spinach), and spices like turmeric might help lower chronic inflammation, which is a contributing factor to pain.

- **Hydration:** Because intervertebral discs are mostly made of water, staying hydrated preserves their pliability and health.

Physical Activity: Low-Impact Spinal Strength Exercises Exercise improves flexibility, develops the muscles that support the spine, and advances general health. Low-impact exercises provide the following advantages while lowering spinal stress:

- Walking improves the muscles in the lower back and increases circulation.

- Because of the buoyancy of the water, swimming is a full-body workout that reduces strain on the spine and joints.

- In order to prevent and relieve back discomfort, yoga and pilates emphasize posture, flexibility, and core strength.

- Stretching tight muscles, such as the hamstrings and hip flexors, on a regular basis will help ease lower back pain.

Best Practices for Preventing Back Pain: Sleep Hygiene

Although getting enough sleep is crucial for maintaining general health and repairing muscles, bad sleeping habits can exacerbate back discomfort. Important procedures consist of:

- **The Best Mattress Choice:** A medium-firm mattress allows for natural spinal alignment while offering support.

Sleeping Position:

- To maintain the lumbar curve, back sleepers should place a pillow beneath their knees.
- A pillow between the knees is beneficial for side sleepers.
- Steer clear of stomach sleeping as it might put tension on the lower back and neck.
- **Regular Sleep Schedule:** Keeping consistent sleep schedules promotes general healing and wellbeing.

Primary Finding: Over time, minor, regular lifestyle changes can greatly improve spine health and avoid back discomfort.

4.2 Changes to the Work Environment

Positioning of Chairs, Desks, and Monitors for Ergonomic Workstations

Back discomfort can be significantly exacerbated by the modern workplace, particularly for people with sedentary jobs. Among the ergonomic adjustments are:

Chair Adjustments:

- Make use of a chair with armrests, lumbar support, and height adjustment.
- Make certain that your feet are flat on the ground or a footrest.
- **Desk Setup:** To lessen neck strain, position the top of the display at eye level or just below.
- To prevent overextension, keep the mouse and keyboard close at hand.
- **Standing Desks:** To relieve strain on the spine, switch between sitting and standing.

Movement and Breaks: The Value of Regular Stretching

Long periods of sitting might cause stiffness by compressing the spinal discs. Frequent pauses can lessen these impacts:

- **Micro-Breaks:** Take a two to three minute walk, stand, and stretch every thirty to sixty minutes.

Include the following stretches in your stretching routine:

- **Seated Spinal Twist:** To increase range of motion and reduce stress.
- To lessen strain on the lower back, stretch your hamstrings.
- **Neck Stretches:** To relieve neck and upper back pain.

One of the main causes of acute back discomfort is incorrect lifting technique, which involves avoiding strain with adequate form. To reduce risk, do the following actions:

1. Make sure the weight is manageable by conducting an assessment of the load. Ask for assistance if required.

2. **Use Your Legs:** Maintain a straight back while bending at the knees and hips.

3. **Hold Close:** To lessen the tension on your spine, keep the object close to your body.

4. **Avoid Twisting**: To keep alignment, turn with your feet rather than your torso.

Primary Finding: Back pain at work can be significantly decreased with an ergonomic workspace and good movement practices.

4.3 Back Pain and Stress

Mind-Body Link: The Effect of Stress on Muscle Tension

Back discomfort is one of the common physical symptoms of stress. This happens because:

- **Muscle Tightening:** Prolonged stress leads to tense muscles, especially in the shoulders, lower back, and neck.

- **Hormonal Impacts:** Stress-induced elevated cortisol levels can cause inflammation and a delayed recovery from strained muscles.

Meditation, Yoga, and Mindfulness as Relaxation Techniques

Back discomfort brought on by stress can be lessened by incorporating relaxation techniques:

- **Yoga:** releases stress and increases spinal flexibility by combining physical postures, breathing techniques, and meditation.

- **Meditation:** Promotes relaxation and lowers stress hormones. Areas of tension can be found and released with the aid of guided body scans.

- **Mindfulness:** By remaining in the now, people can react to pain and stressors more composedly rather than tensely.

Behavioral Cognitive Techniques: Modifying Your Perspective on Pain

A tried-and-true strategy for treating persistent back pain by addressing its psychological component is cognitive behavioral therapy, or CBT:

- **Reframing Thoughts:** Assists patients in changing their negative thoughts such as "This pain will never go away" to positive ones such as "I have tools to manage this pain."

- **Pain Desensitization:** Fear-avoidance tendencies, which frequently exacerbate pain, can be reduced by gradually resuming regular activities.
- **Relaxation Training:** Methods such as progressive muscle relaxation educate people to intentionally relax particular muscle groups.

Primary Finding: One important but frequently disregarded aspect of preventing back pain is stress management. Long-term advantages and substantial relief are possible with mind-body techniques.

A comprehensive strategy that incorporates ergonomic changes, stress reduction, and lifestyle adjustments is needed to prevent back discomfort. Using these techniques improves general health and well-being while reducing the chance of developing back discomfort. People can maintain a healthy spine and live more active, pain-free lives by prioritizing preventive care.

CHAPTER 5

OVERVIEW OF THE MCKENZIE APPROACH

A well-known worldwide strategy for treating back pain and other musculoskeletal conditions is the McKenzie Method, also known as Mechanical Diagnosis and Therapy (MDT). This evidence-based approach, which was created in the 1950s by physiotherapist Robin McKenzie of New Zealand, emphasizes patient empowerment via self-treatment and education. Its focus on locating and treating the underlying mechanical causes of pain rather than only treating its symptoms has made it a pillar of physical therapy.

5.1 The McKenzie Method: What Is It?

Philosophy: Education and Self-Care as Essential Components

The McKenzie Method is based on the fundamental idea that self-treatment is the best way to address the majority of musculoskeletal discomfort. In contrast to many conventional therapies that depend on passive measures like heat therapy or massage, MDT gives patients the tools they need to actively participate in their own healing. The following are the main advantages of this philosophy:

- **Decreased Dependency:** Patients develop self-management skills for their pain, which reduces the frequency of trips to the doctor.

- **Better Results:** Patients can avoid recurrences and preserve long-term spinal health by being aware of their situation.

- **Cost-Effectiveness:** Self-treatment lowers medical expenses by reducing the need for outside therapies.

Centralization and mechanical diagnosis are two important ideas.

Two essential ideas form the basis of the McKenzie Method:

- The concept of centralization During certain movements or activities, discomfort that originates in the spine but radiates to other locations (such as the arms or legs) may retreat back toward the spine. Centralization suggests that the recommended movement is treating the underlying source of the discomfort.

- **The mechanical diagnosis is as follows:** MDT uses a systematic evaluation procedure to categorize pain into mechanical syndromes, which subsequently direct therapy. This method guarantees that interventions are customized to meet the unique needs of each person.

International Recognition: The Reasons Professionals Choose It

Because of its simplicity and efficacy, the McKenzie Method has gained widespread popularity among chiropractors, physical therapists, and other medical practitioners. Its widespread recognition is a result of several factors, including:

- With the support of clinical research, MDT has shown effectiveness in treating a range of musculoskeletal conditions.

- **Adaptability:** Although the technique was first created to address spinal disorders, it has now been modified to treat issues with the extremities, such as knee or shoulder pain.

It is feasible for patients in a variety of contexts, including those with limited access to healthcare, due to its emphasis on self-treatment.

5.2 The Mechanism

Evaluation Procedure: Recognizing Pain and Movement Patterns

The McKenzie Method begins with a thorough evaluation to determine how particular postures or motions affect pain. Important elements of the evaluation consist of:

- **Patient History:** Knowing the origin, location, and kind of pain as well as activities that make symptoms worse or better.

- **Repeated Movement Testing:** As the therapist watches for changes in pain patterns, the patient does a series of movements, such as bending forward or arching backward.

- **Categorization:** Three mechanical syndromes are used to categorize the pain based on the responses:

- Pain from persistently bad posture without structural damage is known as "Postural Syndrome."

- The symptoms of dysfunction syndrome include

pain from damaged or shortened tissues that restricts movement.

- The pain that results from the displacement of spinal components is known as "Derangement Syndrome," and it frequently improves with certain activities.

Exercises: Customized Motions to Reduce Symptoms

The McKenzie Method aims to reduce pain, restore function, and avoid recurrence by prescribing particular exercises based on the patient's classification. Typical workouts consist of:

- **Exercises for Extension:** These exercises, which promote spinal extension to centralize pain and lower disc pressure, are frequently utilized for derangement syndrome.
- Flexion exercises are used to stretch tight tissues and increase mobility in people with certain dysfunction or postural abnormalities.
- **Lateral Motions:** Rotation or side-gliding exercises may be used for patients whose symptoms do not improve with flexion or extension.

Self-Monitoring: Monitoring Development and

Modifying Methods

The McKenzie Method is distinctive in that it relies on self-monitoring, which gives patients the ability to direct their own care. This procedure entails:

- **Pain Journals:** Patients keep a log of their symptoms, noting when they experience more or less pain while engaging in particular activities.

- **Feedback Loops:** Patients keep their therapist informed about their progress on a regular basis, allowing them to modify the workout program as necessary.

The long-term use of these Patients can lower their risk of chronic problems by learning self-assessment strategies that will enable them to manage pain episodes on their own in the future.

5.3 Achievements

Real-World Uses: Testimonials of McKenzie Method Recovery

Real-world success stories provide the best example of the McKenzie Method's efficacy:

- **Case 1: Persistent Lower Back Pain:** Following an

MDT evaluation, a 45-year-old office worker who had been experiencing lower back discomfort for years received relief with extension exercises. She was able to return to her regular activities after the pain subsided after six weeks.

- **Case Study 2: Resolution of Sciatica**: A construction worker received McKenzie-based therapy for radiating leg discomfort. Derangement syndrome was discovered through repeated mobility testing, and the symptoms were alleviated in a matter of weeks with customized workouts.

Results Based on Evidence: Clinical Research Confirming Its Effectiveness

There is strong clinical evidence to support the effectiveness of the McKenzie Method:

- Research has demonstrated that MDT is superior to traditional physical therapy in terms of lowering pain and enhancing function in people with lower back pain.

- **Long-Term Benefits:** Studies show that patients who acquire and apply MDT procedures have fewer pain recurrences than those who only use passive therapies.

The method's empowering and instructive approach is responsible for the consistently high levels of patient satisfaction reported in surveys.

A revolutionary strategy for treating and avoiding musculoskeletal discomfort is the McKenzie Method. Both patients and medical professionals favor it because of its emphasis on patient education, self-treatment, and evidence-based treatments. People can take proactive measures toward long-term spinal health and pain management independence by being aware of its guiding concepts, procedures, and achievements.

CHAPTER 6

Easy Back Health Exercises

Avoiding strain is only one aspect of maintaining a healthy back; regular workouts that promote strength, flexibility, and mobility are also necessary. Easy yet efficient exercises can reduce pain, stop problems later, and enhance spinal health in general. In order to support back health, this chapter examines stretching, core strengthening, and incorporating movement into daily activities.

6.1 Exercises for Stretching

Stretching is essential for back health because it increases circulation, eases tense muscles, and increases flexibility. Maintaining spinal alignment and reducing stiffness can be achieved with a daily stretching regimen.

Hamstring Stretches: Lower Back Tension Reduction

Lower back discomfort can result from tight hamstrings

pulling on the pelvis. Posture is improved and tension is reduced by stretching these muscles.

How to Do It:

1. Put one leg out on the floor and bend the other so that the sole of the foot touches the inside thigh of the outstretched leg.

2. Maintaining a straight back, reach for the outstretched leg's toes.

3. After 20 to 30 seconds of holding the stretch, switch legs.

Benefits include improved posture, increased flexibility, and relief of lower back discomfort.

Encouraging Spinal Flexibility with the Cat-Cow Pose

This yoga-inspired stretch warms up the back muscles and moves the spine.

How to Do It:

1. Take a tabletop position and begin on your hands and knees.

2. Take a deep breath, raise your head and tailbone toward the ceiling, and arch your back (Cow Pose).

3. Pull your tummy toward your spine, tuck your chin, round your back, and exhale (Cat Pose).

4. Slowly and carefully repeat 5–10 times.

Benefits: Increases body awareness, reduces stress, and improves spinal mobility.

Child's Pose: A Calm Method to Reduce Stress

This calming pose encourages relaxation while stretching the thighs, hips, and lower back.

How to Do It:

1. Sit back on your heels while kneeling on the ground.

2. Lower your torso to rest on your thighs after extending your arms forward.

3. Breathe deeply while maintaining the posture for 30 to 60 seconds.

Benefits include reducing lower back strain, promoting spinal flexibility, and calming the mind.

6.2 Strengthening of the Core

Maintaining proper posture and supporting the spine require a strong core. Exercises that strengthen the core lower the chance of injury and improve stability in general.

Planks: Strengthening the Core to Support the Back

A full-body exercise that works the shoulder, back, and abdominal muscles is the plank.

How to Do It:

1. Start by bending your elbows and supporting your weight with your forearms in a push-up stance.

2. Using your core muscles, maintain a straight body from head to heels.

3. As your strength increases, progressively extend the time you hold the position for 20 to 60 seconds.

Enhances balance and stability, strengthens the core, and lessens spinal strain.

Abdominal Muscle Strengthening with Pelvic Tilts

Gentle movements called pelvic tilts help to improve pelvic alignment and strengthen the muscles in the lower abdomen.

How to Do It:

1. Place your feet flat on the floor and bend your knees while lying on your back.

2. Press your lower back against the floor and tighten your abdominal muscles.

3. Release after a few seconds of holding.

4. Do it ten to fifteen times.

Advantages: Reduces lower back discomfort, strengthens the core, and encourages healthy spinal alignment.

Bridges: Improving Spinal and Gluteal Stability

Bridges give the spine the vital support it needs by strengthening the lower back, hamstrings, and glutes.

How to Do It:

1. Place your feet flat on the floor and bend your knees while lying on your back.
2. Raise your hips toward the ceiling so that your shoulders and knees make a straight line.
3. Before descending, hold for a few seconds.
4. Do ten to fifteen reps.

Enhances posture, lessens lower back strain, and increases spinal stability.

6.3 Integration of Daily Movement

Maintaining spinal health requires incorporating activity into your daily routine, particularly if you lead a sedentary lifestyle.

Practices for Standing Desks: Activities to Include While

Working

- Standing workstations facilitate posture and movement adjustments throughout the day. Spinal health can be further enhanced by adding simple workouts.

Easy Motions:

- **Leg Swings:** To improve hip mobility, gently swing each leg forward and backward.
- **Heel Raises:** To increase circulation and develop your calf muscles, raise your heels off the floor.
- **Side Bends:** Gently bend at the waist to stretch your sides.

Prevents stiffness, enhances circulation, and preserves spinal alignment, among other advantages.

Walking's Low-Impact Cardio Benefits for Spine Health

Walking strengthens muscles and improves posture, making it an easy yet effective strategy to promote back health.

Important Advice:

- Every day, try to get in at least 30 minutes of vigorous walking.

- To reduce the amount of tension on the spine, use supportive shoes.

- Keep your head up and shoulders back to maintain proper posture.

Benefits include increased circulation, less stress, and improved spinal flexibility.

Stretch Breaks: Avoiding Stiffness While Sitting for Extended Periods of Time

- Long periods of sitting can cause stiffness and compression of the spine. These effects are offset by regular stretch breaks.

Easy Stretching Ideas:

- **Seated Spinal rotate:** While seated, rotate your torso to one side while maintaining support from the armrest.

- **Neck Stretches:** To release tension in your neck, tilt your head forward and side-to-side.

- **Standing Forward Fold:** To stretch your hamstrings and lower back, stand up and bend forward.

Improves flexibility, eases tense muscles, and encourages improved posture.

Back health can be greatly impacted by easy workouts like stretching, core strengthening, and incorporating regular movement. These techniques not only ease current discomfort but also strengthen resistance to problems in the future. By including these exercises in your regimen, you promote strength, flexibility, and general well-being while making an investment in your long-term spine health.

CHAPTER 7

Effectively treating acute back pain is essential to reducing suffering and keeping the problem from becoming chronic. Although acute back pain, which is frequently brought on by an unexpected accident or strain, can be upsetting, you can speed up your recovery by following the appropriate actions. This chapter provides advice on when to seek expert medical assistance, early recovery exercises, and immediate management techniques.

7.1 Quick Actions

Recovery from acute back pain can be greatly impacted by prompt and suitable action. In order to reduce pain and encourage healing, it is crucial to know when and how to step in.

Applying Heat and Ice: When and How to Do It

- One of the simplest yet most successful first-line therapies for acute back pain is the administration of heat or ice. Depending on the type and time of the pain, each offers unique advantages.
- **Ice Therapy:** To minimize swelling and inflammation, it is best applied within the first 24 to 48 hours following an injury.
- Every one to two hours, apply an ice pack wrapped in a thin towel to the painful area for 15 to 20 minutes.
- To avoid frostbite, do not apply ice straight to the skin.
- It works well for ailments including strained muscles or wounds that have obvious edema.
- **Heat Therapy:** Beneficial 48 hours after the injury, or after the initial inflammation has subsided.
- Spend 15 to 20 minutes at a time with a heated cloth or heating pad.
- Reduces muscular stiffness, increases blood flow, and eases the symptoms of chronic pain.
- Perfect for discomfort caused by muscle spasms or stiffness.

Medications Over-the-Counter for Temporary Pain Relief

Over-the-counter (OTC) drugs may be useful for providing instant pain relief:

- **Nonsteroidal Anti-Inflammatory Drugs (NSAIDs):** Pain and inflammation are lessened by drugs such as naproxen or ibuprofen.
- **Acetaminophen:** A substitute for people unable to take NSAIDs, although it mainly treats pain instead of inflammation.

Warnings: Always take your drugs as prescribed, and if you take additional medications or have underlying medical concerns, speak with your doctor.

Soft Motions: The Value of Steering Clear of Total Rest

Long-term immobility can exacerbate back pain, even if resting may seem like the body's natural reaction to it:

- Mild exercises promote healing by preserving blood flow to the wounded area.
- Steer clear of activities like walking or stretching that make the pain worse while still allowing for light movement.
- Long-term bed rest can cause weakness, stiffness,

and a prolonged recovery period.

7.2 Initial Recuperation Activities

Including safe and mild activities in your regimen when the initial pain starts to go away might hasten recovery and stop recurrence.

Realigning Your Posture: Easy Methods to Lessen Stress

- Maintaining good posture is essential for reducing back discomfort. The spine and surrounding muscles are subjected to excessive strain when there is misalignment.
- Maintain a straight posture when standing, with your head in line with your spine, your shoulders back, and your weight evenly balanced on both feet.
- **Seated Posture:** Place your feet flat on the floor and support your back. Steer clear of prolonged forward tilting or slouching.
- **Sleeping Posture:** Sleep on your side or back with a pillow between your legs or beneath your knees, and use a supportive mattress.

Breathing Methods: Using Relaxation to Reduce Pain

Breathing exercises that promote relaxation and ease tense muscles might assist manage pain:

Breathing Diaphragmatically:

1. Bend your knees and lie on your back.

2. Put your hands on your abdomen and chest, respectively.

3. Let your belly rise as you take a deep breath through your nostrils.

4. Slowly exhale through your mouth while concentrating on letting your muscles relax.

5. Continue for five to ten minutes.

Reduces stress, lessens the impression of pain, and encourages general relaxation.

Light Activities: Safely Returning to Daily Tasks

Normal function is restored and stiffness is avoided by gradually reintroducing everyday activities:

- **Walking:** As your pain goes away, increase the length and distance of your walks from short, easy ones.

- To preserve flexibility, use mild stretches such as the

knee-to-chest stretch or the Cat-Cow pose.

- **Avoid Overexertion:** Pay attention to your body's cues and cease activities that cause sudden pain.

7.3 Knowing When to Get Medical Assistance

Acute back pain usually goes away with self-care, but some symptoms need to be treated right away. By identifying these symptoms, consequences can be avoided and prompt intervention is ensured.

Red Flags: Signs That Need to Be Addressed Immediately

Certain symptoms should not be disregarded as they may point to a more serious underlying condition:

- Pain that is severe or getting worse in spite of self-care techniques.
- Leg weakness or numbness, particularly if it interferes with walking.
- Loss of control over one's bowels or bladder, which could be a sign of cauda equina syndrome.
- A history of malignancy, unexplained weight loss, or pain coupled with a fever.

- Chronic pain following a catastrophic injury, like an accident or fall.

Diagnostic Instruments: Imaging and Examination for Severe Situations

Diagnostic tools assist in determining the cause when warning signs are present or pain continues:

- **X-rays:** Beneficial for detecting spine fractures or structural anomalies.
- **MRI or CT Scans:** Offer fine-grained pictures of soft tissues, such as muscles, discs, and nerves.
- **Electromyography (EMG):** Evaluates nerve function and detects possible injury to the nerves.
- **Blood Tests:** Disqualify inflammatory diseases or infections.

Expert Interventions: When Conventional Approaches Don't Work

Experts may suggest cutting-edge therapies in circumstances that are severe or unresponsive:

- **Physical therapy:** An organized regimen to regain function, strength, and mobility.
- **Injections:** Injections of corticosteroids decrease

inflammation in particular regions of the spine.

- **Surgical Options:** In rare instances, spinal stenosis, fractures, or herniated discs may require surgery.

A balanced strategy is essential for acute back pain, which includes prompt medical attention, progressive rehabilitation activities, and, if necessary, expert evaluation. You may confidently handle acute bouts while lowering the chance of long-term problems by knowing how to effectively manage pain and identifying warning indications. The basis for long-term spinal health and resilience is laid by making the right investments in care during the acute phase.

CHAPTER 8

The Impact of Postural Stress

In today's world, postural stress is a common problem that is frequently brought on by extended sitting, bad standing habits, and repeated motions. Musculoskeletal abnormalities, chronic health problems, and severe discomfort can all result from poor posture. Maintaining general well being requires knowing the origins of postural stress and using techniques to deal with it.

8.1 Postural Stress Science

Long-term maintenance of less-than-ideal postures causes postural stress, which puts excessive strain on the musculoskeletal system. Here is a detailed examination of the ways in which various behaviors and circumstances contribute to this phenomena.

Long-Term Sitting Problems: Impact on Spinal

Alignment

Long periods of sitting, particularly with bad posture, alter the spine's natural curvature:

- **Forward Head Posture:** The head shifts forward when one leans near a screen, putting more strain on the cervical spine.

- **Rounded Shoulders:** Slouching while seated causes the chest to constrict and the back muscles to weaken, which leads to an unbalanced posture.

- **Lower Back Compression:** Excessive lumbar strain from poor chair support might result in herniated discs.

These issues are made worse by modern lives, since many people spend hours slumped over mobile devices or at computers.

Standing Issues: Difficulties from Inappropriate Footwear or Posture

Inappropriate footwear and improper standing posture both lead to postural stress:

- **Locked Knees:** When standing with your knees hyperextended, your weight is incorrectly transferred to your lower back.

- **Flat Feet:** Insufficient arch support puts more strain on the knees and spine.
- **High Heels:** High heels cause the lower back to overarch and the pelvis to lean forward, changing the alignment of the body.

Repeated Stress: Minor Behaviors Resulting in Major Issues

Cumulative stress injuries can result from repetitive motions, even minor ones:

- **Micro-Movements:** Constantly reaching for objects, typing, or using a mouse can cause wrist, shoulder, and neck discomfort.
- **Imbalanced Loads:** Muscle distribution and spinal alignment are impacted by carrying big loads or often slanting to one side.
- **Cumulative Effects:** These behaviors eventually lead to joint damage, muscle imbalances, and persistent discomfort.

8.2 Techniques for Improving Posture

Consistent practice, the right equipment, and deliberate effort are all necessary to improve posture. Postural stress can be considerably decreased by concentrating on alignment when standing, sitting, and sleeping.

Alignment and Balance Tips for Standing Posture

Standing with the right alignment eases the strain on the spine and improves muscular balance.

- **Head Position:** Avoid protruding your head forward and maintain it level with your shoulders.

- **Shoulders and Chest:** Without overdoing it, expand your chest a little and relax your shoulders.

- **Pelvis and Spine:** Prevent excessive forward or backward tilting to maintain a neutral pelvis. In order to maintain this posture, contract your core muscles.

Place your feet shoulder-width apart and balance your weight equally on both of them.

Sitting Posture: Appropriate Chair Adjustments and Support

Maintaining optimal sitting posture helps to protect the natural curves of the spine and avoid strain:

- **Chair Height:** Set your chair so that your knees are at a 90-degree angle and your feet are flat on the floor.

- To maintain lower back support, choose a chair with a curved backrest or install a lumbar roll.

- When typing, keep your arms close to your body, elbows bent at a 90-degree angle, and wrists straight.

- **Screen Position:** To prevent neck strain, place your screen at eye level.

Selecting the appropriate mattress and position for sleeping is crucial for maintaining spinal health.

- **Choosing a Mattress:** Select a mattress that is medium-firm enough to accommodate your spine's natural curvature.

Positions for Sleeping:

- Back Sleepers: To lessen the tension on your lower back, place a pillow beneath your knees.

- Side sleepers: To maintain hip alignment, place a pillow between your knees.

- Steer clear of stomach sleeping since it frequently twists the neck in an awkward way.

8.3 Posture-Improving Tools

Using ergonomic equipment can improve posture and reduce musculoskeletal strain.

Features to Consider in Ergonomic Chairs

The purpose of ergonomic chairs is to promote optimal body alignment and reduce pain from extended sitting:

- With its adjustable height, you can keep your knees at a 90-degree angle and place your feet flat on the floor.

- **Lumbar Support:** Maintains the natural curve of the spine by offering sufficient lower back support.

- With a small space between the back of your knees and the chair edge, the seat's depth and width guarantee that your thighs are properly supported.

The tilt mechanism reduces stiffness by encouraging dynamic sitting and movement.

Lumbar Support Equipment: Choices to Improve Comfort

Ordinary chairs can be converted into back-friendly seating solutions with the help of portable lumbar supports:

- The lumbar area is specifically supported by the contoured contours of the foam cushions.

- **Inflatable Supports:** Firmness can be changed for individualized comfort.

- Chairs with integrated lumbar support for ongoing alignment are known as "integrated chair designs."

Wearable Posture Trainers: Advantages and Drawbacks

Wearable technology offers mild reminders to assist people improve their postural awareness:

- **How They Operate**: In order to promote realignment, these gadgets usually vibrate when the wearer slouches.

- Improved awareness of posture throughout the day is one of the benefits.

- It's simple to use and incorporate into everyday activities.

Restrictions:

- Short-term fixes that need regular application to have long-term effects.

- If not combined with core-strengthening activities, it is less effective.

If untreated, postural stress can result in long-term musculoskeletal problems and persistent discomfort. However, you may reduce stress and support spinal health by being aware of its science, using ergonomic tools, and putting posture modification practices into practice. Conscious changes in sleeping, sitting, and standing patterns, along with the use of assistive technology, provide the groundwork for improved posture and general health. Putting money into these techniques guarantees a better quality of life in addition to a healthier spine.

CHAPTER 9

A variety of individualized treatments are frequently used to effectively manage back pain. To manage pain and enhance quality of life, it is essential to comprehend the available solutions, which range from prescription drugs to activity management and complementary therapies. In order to assist you in making well-informed judgments regarding the treatment of back pain, this chapter examines the variety of possible therapies, their uses, and their drawbacks.

9.1 Back Pain Medicines

Medications are essential for treating back pain because they reduce inflammation and discomfort. But using them necessitates carefully weighing the hazards, dosage, and effectiveness.

Over-the-Counter Choices: The Function of NSAIDs

For mild to severe back pain, non-steroidal anti-inflammatory medications (NSAIDs) are frequently the first line of treatment:

- NSAIDs, such as naproxen and ibuprofen, function by decreasing inflammation, which is frequently a major cause of pain.

- **Accessibility:** These drugs are generally accessible without a prescription and work well to temporarily relieve pain from minor injuries or strained muscles.

- **Disclaimers:** Extended usage of NSAIDs should be used with caution since it may result in gastrointestinal problems, such as ulcers.

Prescription Drugs: When More Powerful Choices Are Required

Healthcare professionals may suggest prescription drugs for more severe or chronic back pain:

- Muscle relaxants, which assist ease muscle tension but can make you sleepy, are frequently used for severe pain and muscle spasms.

- **Opioids:** Opioids like oxycodone or hydrocodone, which are reserved for extreme pain, offer powerful pain relief but come with a high risk of addiction and dependence.

- Off-label, some antidepressants, like amitriptyline, are used to treat chronic back pain, particularly when nerve pain is present.

Dangers and Adverse Reactions: Handling Pain Effectively

- Despite their effectiveness, drugs can have negative side effects.

- Risks associated with NSAIDs include kidney strain, cardiovascular hazards, and gastrointestinal discomfort.

- **Opioids:** Constipation, nausea, and vertigo, as well as a high risk of reliance.

- **Overall Instructions:** Never take more medication than is advised, and always get advice from a healthcare professional to determine the right dosage.

9.2 Activity and Rest in Bed

Back pain used to often be treated with prolonged bed

rest. However, recent studies have demonstrated that too much sleep can worsen symptoms and impede recovery.

The Reasons Bed Rest Is No Longer Suggested: Contemporary Knowledge

Extended bed rest is no longer advised for a number of reasons:

- **muscular Weakness:** Prolonged immobility causes muscular atrophy, which lessens the spine's support.
- **Stiffness:** Inactivity can cause feelings of helplessness, worry, and sadness, which can intensify the impression of pain.
- **Psychological Impact:** Inactivity can exaccrbate joint stiffness, making rehabilitation more challenging.

Gradual Activity Resumption: Safely Re-Engaging with Daily Life

Recovery depends on a supervised return to regular activities:

- **Low-Impact Movements:** To keep circulation and flexibility, start with mild cxcrcises like walking.
- **Prevent Overexertion:** Increase exercise lcvcls

gradually without enduring excruciating pain.

- **Adhere to Professional Advice:** To guarantee safe advancement, physical therapists can design customized workout regimens.

Listening to Your Body: Juggling Movement and Rest

Finding the ideal balance between movement and rest is crucial:

- **Rest Periods:** Resting for brief periods of time might help, particularly while experiencing severe pain.

- **Active Recovery:** To maintain muscular engagement, include low-impact workouts or gentle stretching.

- **Body Signals:** Keep an eye out for signs of weariness and pain, and use them to modify your level of exercise.

9.3 Alternative Medicine

For back pain alleviation, many people use complementary therapies in addition to traditional treatments. Some are still more debatable, even if there is substantial data to support their efficacy.

Acupuncture: Proof of Its Efficiency

Thin needles are inserted into particular body sites during acupuncture, an ancient Chinese medical procedure:

- **Pain Modulation:** Research indicates that acupuncture may lessen inflammation and promote the body's natural analgesics, endorphins, to be released.

- **Evidence:** A growing amount of studies suggests that acupuncture may help with persistent back pain, particularly when used in conjunction with other therapies.

- **Practical Considerations:** To lower the risk of infection, be sure the practitioner is licensed and employs sterile procedures.

Chiropractic Care: Benefits and Controversies

Spinal manipulation is the main goal of chiropractic adjustments in order to enhance alignment and reduce pain:

- Many patients, especially those with mechanical problems like displaced vertebrae, claim instant alleviation from back discomfort.

- **Disputes:** Critics contend that diseases like nerve compression and ruptured discs are less effectively treated by chiropractic care. Sometimes, misaligned modifications might make discomfort worse.

- **The process of choosing a practitioner:** Give your symptoms and medical history to a chiropractor who has experience treating back pain.

Massage Therapy: Addressing Pain and Muscle Tension

Enhancing circulation and reducing muscle tension are two benefits of massage therapy that can reduce pain:

Techniques:

- **Swedish Massage:** Calm methods to ease tense muscles.

- To alleviate deeper muscular knots, apply focused pressure during a deep tissue massage.

- Targeting certain muscular tension points is the goal of trigger point therapy.

- The benefits of massage include lowering cortisol levels, encouraging relaxation, and improving general wellbeing.

- Massage is useful for treating muscle soreness, but it

might not be able to address structural or nerve-related problems.

Back pain management frequently calls for a multimodal strategy. Although medications might offer instant relief, their usage should be cautious and guided by a physician. Similar to this, healing is aided and deconditioning is avoided by striking a balance between rest and a gradual return to exercise. Additional options for treatment are provided by complementary therapies like massage, acupuncture, and chiropractic adjustments, especially when incorporated into a larger pain management strategy. People can significantly improve their back health and general quality of life by being aware of and making sensible use of these options and cures.

CHAPTER 10

LIVING A PAIN-FREE BACK LIFESTYLE

A pain-free back is frequently the consequence of continuous lifestyle choices rather than merely temporary fixes or medical procedures. Back pain can be considerably decreased while enhancing general wellness by forming routines that promote spinal health and attending to the interrelated elements of physical and mental health. This chapter explores long-term fitness regimens, everyday routines, and the critical role that mental and emotional well-being play in maintaining a healthy back.

10.1 Routines

Spinal health is impacted by daily activities over time. You may improve your quality of life and avoid back discomfort by forming mindful, health-promoting habits.

Remaining Active: The Value of Consistent Movement

Back discomfort is primarily caused by sedentary lifestyles. Frequent exercise is beneficial:

- By keeping muscles and ligaments flexible, movement lowers the chance of strain or stiffness.

- **Improve Circulation:** Active bodies guarantee sufficient blood flow to spinal discs, supplying the nutrients and oxygen required for upkeep and repair.

- **Prevent Deconditioning:** Inactivity can cause the muscles that support the spine to weaken, which increases the risk of injury and causes poor posture.

Make movement a part of your day by taking quick walks when you have time off from work.

- Every hour, especially if you spend a lot of time sitting down, stretch your body.

- Take part in low-impact exercises like swimming or cycling to maintain the health of your spine.

Hydration: Promoting Disc Health with Appropriate Water Consumption

Hydration is essential for the flexibility and shock-absorbing qualities of spinal discs, which serve as cushions between vertebrae:

- **Discs' Water Content:** About 70–90% of healthy discs are composed of water. Reduced disc height and function due to dehydration might make a person more prone to discomfort and injury.

- **Daily Hydration Objectives:** Aim for 8–10 glasses of water per day, taking climate and activity levels into account.

- **Practical Advice:** Keep a bottle of water close at hand, consume foods high in water, such as fruits and vegetables, and refrain from drinking too much alcohol or caffeine, as these substances can cause dehydration.

Posture Checks: Regular Self-Evaluation During the Day

Over time, poor posture can cause pain by putting tension on the spine and surrounding muscles. It's critical to regularly assess your posture:

- Make sure your feet are flat on the floor, your shoulders are relaxed, and your back is straight as you sit. For more comfort, use lumbar support.

- Maintain a balanced weight distribution on both feet, a modest bend in your knees, and a head that is in line with your spine when standing.

- Utilization of Technology: Use ergonomic accessories and place screens at eye level to prevent stooping over them.

Make a note to check your posture at regular intervals during the day, particularly when performing longer duties like sitting at a computer.

10.2 Extended Exercise Programs

One of the best strategies to support a back free of discomfort is to include structured exercise in your regimen. Exercise promotes overall spinal health, increases flexibility, and strengthens muscles.

Enhancing Core Strength and Flexibility with Yoga and Pilates

There are several advantages to these low-impact back health practices:

- The Cat-Cow and Downward Dog are two yoga positions that increase spinal flexibility.
- Encourages relaxation, which lessens stress-related

muscle tension.

- The goal of Pilates is to strengthen the core, which is essential for maintaining spinal stability.

- Incorporates workouts that target the deep abdominal and pelvic muscles, including the Plank or Bridge.

These exercises are perfect for people of all fitness levels since they place an emphasis on precise alignment and controlled movements.

Weight Training: Strengthening the Spine with Muscle"
A strong support system is produced by strengthening the muscles that surround the spine:

- Exercises like leg raises and crunches help strengthen the core muscles, which are one of the main areas to focus on.

- **Back Muscles:** The erector spinae and latissimus dorsi are great muscles to train with rows and deadlifts.

- **Glutes:** Squats and lunges improve pelvic and lower back stability.

- **Safe Practices:** To prevent injuries, start with

reasonable weights, use appropriate form, and think about working with a trainer.

The Benefits of Aerobic Exercise for Stress Reduction and General Health Promotion

Cardiovascular workouts indirectly enhance spinal health by enhancing circulation, endurance, and general health:

- Walking is a low-impact activity that encourages flexibility and natural spinal mobility.
- **Swimming:** Offers a full-body workout while easing joint pressure.
- **Cycling:** Provides cardiovascular advantages, but make sure your bike is ergonomically sound to prevent back pain.

For long-lasting effects, it is important to be consistent and perform aerobic exercises at least three to five times per week.

10.3 Emotional and Mental Wellbeing

Because the mind and body are inextricably linked, back pain can be a physical manifestation of stress or emotional difficulties. Preventing and managing back pain requires addressing mental and emotional well-being.

Mind-Body Link: The Effect of Stress on Physical Pain

Cortisol, a hormone that can exacerbate inflammation and muscle tension, is released in response to stress:

- **Muscle Tightness:** Prolonged stress frequently causes tightness in the shoulders, lower back, and neck.
- **Perception of Pain:** Stress can increase sensitivity to pain, exacerbating preexisting discomfort.

These bodily impacts can be lessened by implementing stress-management techniques:

- Reduce stress by practicing mindfulness exercises like meditation.
- To encourage relaxation, including physical exercises like tai chi or yoga.

Cognitive-Behavioral Therapy as a Treatment Option for Chronic Pain

A psychological technique called cognitive-behavioral therapy (CBT) assists people in altering how they perceive pain:

- **Reframing Thoughts:** Cognitive behavioral therapy (CBT) helps people recognize and change pain-related negative thought patterns.

- **Coping Strategies:** Patients acquire mental toughness, pacing, and relaxation techniques.

- **Effectiveness Evidence:** According to studies, cognitive behavioral therapy (CBT) can greatly enhance quality of life and lessen the severity of chronic pain.

Meditation and Journaling: Instruments for Emotional Processing

Emotional tension can be released through expressive practices like journaling and meditation:

- **Journaling:** Putting thoughts and feelings on paper might help you find patterns and stressors that might be causing your pain.

- Frequent meditation practice lowers stress hormones, increases mental clarity, and encourages relaxation.

- **Combining Techniques:** Begin by keeping a gratitude diary to help you concentrate on the good things in life, and then take a quick break to meditate to help you decompress.

It takes a comprehensive strategy that incorporates daily routines, organized exercise, and mental health to create a lifestyle focused on back pain that goes beyond simple physical changes. You lay the groundwork for spinal health by continuing to be active, drinking enough water, and paying attention to your posture. While cardiovascular exercises improve general health, long-term fitness regimens like yoga, pilates, and weight training fortify your body's support structure. Lastly, treating mental and emotional well-being with mindfulness exercises, counseling, and stress management guarantees that you're addressing back pain from all sides.

Having a pain-free back is a lifelong choice, not simply a goal. One deliberate decision at a time, you're investing in your long-term health by adopting these tactics.

ABOUT THE AUTHOR

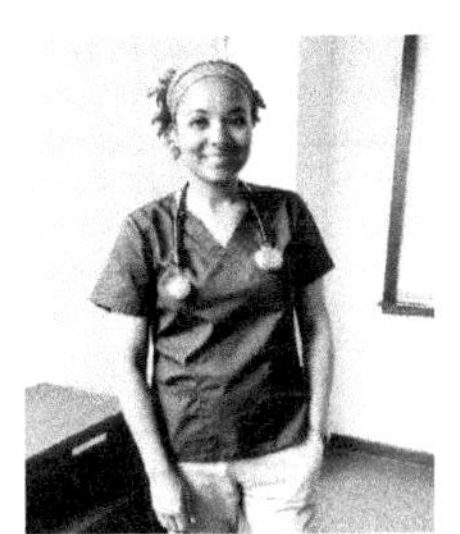

Harmony Royce is a dedicated healthcare worker who has a strong interest in holistic wellness. Harmony's extensive history in various aspects of health and wellness provides her with a wealth of knowledge and expertise that she can utilize in her writing and professional endeavors.

Harmony is a talented author who crafts thought-provoking books that inspire readers to have well-rounded, balanced lives. She writes about a variety of health-related topics, such as diet, exercise, mental health, and mindfulness. Her approachable writing style combines practical guidance with evidence-based research to make complex health concepts approachable and engaging for readers of all ages.

Harmony actively promotes the benefits of holistic health through writing, community workshops, and internet forums. Her mission is to educate and inspire people about the transformative power of self care and healthy lifestyle choices.